How to Save a Life

HEALING POWER OF POETRY

Barbara Loeb, MD

Artwork of Judy "Salsa" Loeb

Published By Mind2Heal
P.O Box 431
Downers Grove, IL 60515
Mind2Heal.com

ISBN- Paperback- 978-1-7378524-0-7

Printed in the United States of America

In writing and publishing this book, neither the author nor publisher are
engaged in rendering professional medical services or providing medical
advice to the individual reader. The ideas, practices and suggestions
contained in this book are not intended to diagnose, treat, prevent, or
cure any disease. They are not intended to substitute for consulting your
physician or other health care provider. If you have any medical or health
concerns or questions, please consult your physician or other qualified
healthcare provider. Neither the author nor the publisher shall be liable
or responsible for any damages or losses allegedly arising from the
information or suggestions in this book.

Cover: Artwork of Judy "Salsa" Loeb

How to Save a Life

To all Generations

Judy "Salsa" Loeb
Morris Loeb
& Antionette Goetschel,
who grounded me.

Rachael, Janeen, Amy, Joseph, Sarah Rose
Dominic, Carter, Max, Gavin,
Mikyal, Finley, Zeke, Dean,
Aidan, Ariya & Knox,
who I aspire to ground.

Danny, partner on all of my adventures.

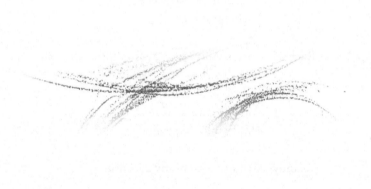

Time of Words

When those feelings begin,
tears pour from within,
and the words come right out,
in a silent shout,
and they slide from the tongue,
fall off the lips,
flow from the pen so free—

This is the time of words,
and life's in perfect harmony.

Barbara Loeb 1968

Table of Contents

Prologue

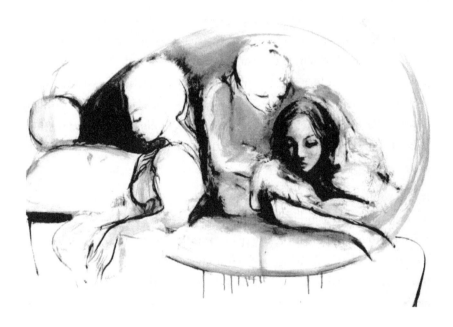

Those who are passionate about helping and healing others often lose sight of their own need for nurturing. The truth is, every human needs self-care. Unrecognized, this can leave us de-energized, prevent flourishing, and even block joy. For most of my life, I was such an individual. Caught up in my role as a physician, mother, partner, and leader; I failed to acknowledge that part of me had been left unattended. This failure to fortify my internal resources made my life much more difficult. I often felt unsupported, stifled with the heaviness of pushing a large boulder, like Sisyphus, up a steep hill. I have seen this same challenge in many of my colleagues. For physicians, just like for so many others in healthcare, there is a secret oath of infallibility that we feel we must uphold. This is paired with an unconscious denial of the importance of self-care.

In my younger years, I used to write almost daily. I wrote everything from poetry, short stories and journals to research papers, and essays. I found that writing provided me with a sanctuary from the stress of my early life, as I struggled with the challenges of becoming of age. In a 40-year career in healthcare, that was gradually lost. I didn't take the time to stop, reflect, celebrate my life, or nurture my soul.

In the fall of 2019, my career was unexpectedly pushed off course. By winter I felt increasingly unsettled. In retrospect this was only choppy water compared to the tidal wave the world would soon face. Still, I felt completely uprooted and directionless. In an attempt to ground myself, I decided to attend a mindfulness retreat at the Deer Park Monastery in Escondido, California. This was a peaceful place of reflection started by the Zen Master Thich Nhat Hanh. The gathering focused on connecting and preserving Mother Earth. The participants came from all parts of the country. We each brought some local soil which we ceremonially mixed in a gigantic bottle. This ritual was followed by a discussion of the impermanence of our individual identities.

The monastic asked the members present to raise their hands if they could recall the names and faces of their parents. Almost all hands went up. When she asked about grandparents, most hands remained raised. Next, she asked about great-grandparents, and the majority of hands went down. When she got to great-great-grandparents, only a few raised hands were left. The point is that in a hundred years from now, our names, faces and voices will be unknown. Whereas, if we don't destroy it, the Earth, from which we all came and will return to, will remain. Our identities which we considered so important will blend into one. Even knowing this to be true, a part of me wanted to reach out to future generations to leave a legacy, a message. This prompted me to write the first poem in this collection "To All Generations with Love." This marked the first phase of my journey.

In March 2020, the unanticipated tsunami hit. The spread of infections caused by *SARS-CoV-2, COVID-19*, was declared a worldwide pandemic. Its widespread impact added another layer of complexity on top of my already existing challenges. With loss, death, restrictions, and confusion, I turned more intensely to my mindfulness practice, spending time communing with nature as a way to deal with the upheaval happening all around. This heralded in the second phase of my journey. Sitting in meditation, I turned inward, fearlessly reflecting on both my inner and outer worlds: Who am I? Where do I belong? What really matters? How can I not only survive but thrive? Traveling along this path, a need for creativity and self-expression emerged.

My morning ritual became mindfully sitting and then writing poetry. Pausing, I focused on noticing details of my surroundings and the sensations, thoughts, and feelings that arose. This became a way to turn my attention from outward difficulties to inward reflection. Without moving, I was able to travel deep into my soul. I began to experience nature, people, and life in a completely different way.

This newly found perspective and mode of self-expression was healing. I was able to lean into my distress, acknowledge it, and without fighting back, soften the edge. Energized, and renewed, I became better equipped to face barriers with calm and clarity. Writing was my way to set free what wanted to be expressed. It was like I had rubbed Aladdin's lamp and let out a healing genie. I recognized the natural wisdom we all possess, the importance of living with love in every moment and the immeasurable value of life "just as it is." This marked the final phase of my journey. I found my way to healing and back home.

I share these poems as an invitation to you, the reader, to come along and find your own journey. Writing is healing during difficult times. It allows our souls to open and our spirits to expand. We realize our natural wisdom and as we grow, our creativity flourishes. We feel more grounded and connected, ultimately leaving room for greater joy.

This is of critical importance to all of us as we work to care for others and need tools to care for ourselves. Whether you are in healthcare (as I was in my career) or a caretaker in another setting, or simply express care in the numerous ways we humans attend to each other, this is for you. I hope you enjoy sharing the journey.

Introduction

Writing *"How to Save a Life: Healing Power of Poetry"* saved *my* life from going into a downward spiral during those dark pandemic months—a time that was filled with loss and challenges. A time when I was unable to hold my father's hand as he passed away in isolation on his 90th birthday. When I saw my mother-in-law die after a long struggle with dementia. When my husband and I put on our masks and rushed across the country to our daughter's side to help after a near fatal accident left our 2-year-old grandson temporarily paralyzed.

This collection of poems is a product of my healing expedition during these trying times. It is for past, present, and future generations of life travelers. It is for caregivers who may have lost touch with their need for self-care and creativity while focusing on others.

The chapters mark the phases of my journey, and the individual poems reflect what was revealed to me along the way with themes of the current times sprinkled in. The illustrations are taken from the artwork of my late mother Judy "Salsa" Loeb and add to the timeless legacy of the volume.

Chapter One – *Grounding,* reflections on our roots, past generations and ancestors who ground us into the future.

Chapter Two – *Awakening,* celebrating the morning, renewal, possibilities, new times, heralding in change.

Chapter Three - *Noticing,* appreciating, and experiencing the richness of all things. Seeing nature and life through new eyes.

Chapter Four – *Transforming,* searching deeper to discover one's true self.

Chapter Five – *Healing,* connecting with the healing energy that supports, nurtures, and mends us.

Epilogue - Humanity's Spring, marks the exuberant release as the pandemic burden first lightened, with awareness emerging.

Appendix contains further details on the individual poems.

As you the reader, follow my journey, I hope you are inspired to find your way back home with energy, creativity, and healing.

Chapter One

Grounding

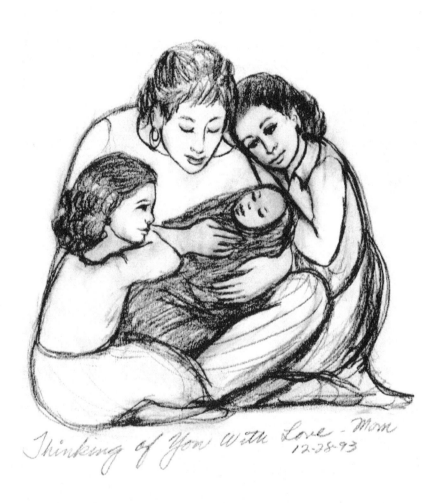

Thinking of You With Love - Mom
12-28-93

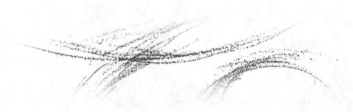

To All Generations with Love

Know that I am always with you.
I am the wind that refreshes you,
　　　　the sand, the water, the rocks and even the asphalt.

In the morning, I am the smile on your lips when you awaken.
In the evening, I am the blanket that tucks you in as you fall asleep.

I am the food nourishing and energizing you,
　　　　the seasoning that makes it so tasty,
　　　　the water that quenches your thirst.

Whether you're at school, work, or home,
　　　　I am the "congratulations" for a job well done,
　　　　the cheers of the crowd, the applause, the simple thank you.

I am the loving kiss on your brow,
　　　　the embrace that holds you when you are frightened or lonely,
　　　　the tissue that dries tears of both sadness and joy.

I am the happiness you feel when your heart opens,
　　　　when you see the beauty that surrounds you,
　　　　when you are moved to extend a helping hand.

You are never alone!

I am there during every moment, every breath, every step,
　　　　every joy or sorrow, every failure, and every success.

To know my presence, close your eyes and feel me within you—
I'm always there—
　　　　even when you can no longer hear my voice or know my face,
　　　　I'll remain a loving part of you forever.

Judy Salsa's Tranquility Garden
(For my mom)

As I stepped into her garden
among yellow daffodils in bloom,
I could hear her last words:
"I'm good.... Everything is resolved. I'm at peace."
They were spoken with great calm and clarity,
as if she knew they'd be the last words we'd share.

I lit the sage taken from my pocket,
waving it in the air.
The smoky sweet aroma was reminiscent
of the scent of cigarettes and perfume,
which in life, heralded her arrival.
I bent down to pick up a cigarette butt.
I turned around as if she were next to me.

She was not your typical mother
Her presence always aroused your senses.
She illuminated every room:
red lipstick,
wild flaxen hair,
pendent earrings twinkling,
rings on every finger,
multicolored bracelets,
miniskirts and four-inch heels,
highlighting her shapely legs.

Her steps produced a clicking vibration
as she moved to greet you.
Her energy pushing you beyond
her external coverings, to reveal her deeper soul.

Eclectic, artistic, spiritual, intuitive,
She took your hand,
opening a window to limitless beauty.

Like the Tarot Empress,
she was a nurturer of creativity—
her deck still wrapped with a silk cloth,
inside a wooden box in my nightstand drawer.

Her life was an incredibly challenging journey.
She was a single mom,
struggling to raise two children,
yet she always found space
to share her numerous gifts with the world;
Paintings, drawings, sculptures,
Jungian teachings of the collective unconscious,
ways to heal oneself and elevate humanity.

In Salsa, she moved with a Zen grace and presence.
She enriched my life in ways I am only beginning to realize.
She left this earth in peace.
While, like the name of her favorite perfume,
she left behind her essence,
An Impression of Eternity.

May her everlasting presence
bring all who enter this tranquility garden,
whether in person or in spirit,
a sense of calm, clarity, and peace.

May they be safe, supported and connected.
May all people, near or distant, enter their own tranquility garden
and find all that they seek to fulfill in their lives.

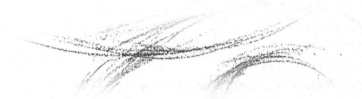

The Red Cardinal

(For my dad)

The red cardinal is perched
on a barren bush outside my window.

Tilting his head,
he beckons me to come near.
As I approach,
he turns and flies away.

Who are you my brightly plumed friend?
A soon-to-depart-spirit
coming to comfort me
and whisper: *"Time to let go."*

Or one already set free,
gently uttering: *"You're not alone."*

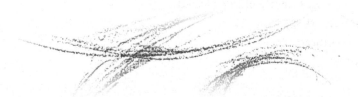

The Red Cardinal Returns

Buried in the grass,
the red cardinal pops out to say:
"Howdy! You thought I'd gone,
but I haven't and I won't.
When you have lost faith,
when you least expect me,
I will appear to reassure you
that it will be okay."

We all have a red cardinal watching over us.
Look out into the distance,
and you will find yours.

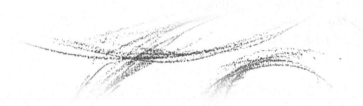

Coming Home
(For Grandma Toni)

The Lady in Purple
stands by the door.
Smiling,
she steps across the threshold.

Clouds clearing,
she rises on lavender butterfly wings,
shimmering as she enters the crimson sky.

Gazing back her face is soft.
Pain and fear gone,
peaceful, shining.

Her delicate body dancing,
fluttering, flitting, floating free,
on her final journey,
Home.

We Never Know

I
When you step outside the door,
pause,
look back,
smile and send love.
You never know
when it will be the last time
you see that face,
that smile.
You never know
when you will last kiss that cheek,
and whisper "I love you."

II
Life is fragile,
she comes, she goes in her own time.
She exits when the gate opens and heaven greets her,
God extending loving arms.
The gate closes, and then she is gone.

III
Darling gently close your eyes,
feel the kiss,
hear the words, "I love you, mom."
Feel peace within your soul,
enfolded in love forever.

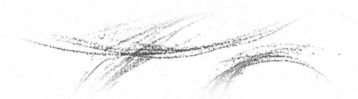

Chapter Two

Awakening

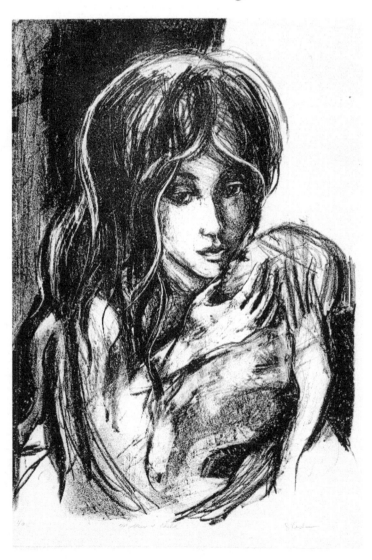

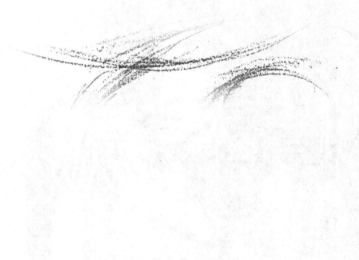

Never-ending Circle

I gave you life.
You gave me life.
We merge into this life.

You brought forth new life.
We join together.

The circle, at first small,
widens, spirals, unwinds.
It fills the room,
crosses the country,
encircles the Earth,
spans the universe.

We ride the curves,
whirl, twist and turn,
then come to rest in the center.
Hand in hand,
the cord of love connects us,
through infinite space and time.

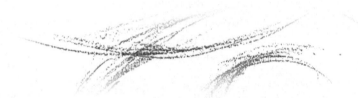

This Morning

Opening my eyes from dreaming,
it's a new day.
At first, I thought *it's yesterday,*
but brush those thoughts away.

Opening my eyes,
I feel the dry air,
I see the bright sun—
my senses awaken.

It's today!

Closing my eyes,
and opening them up again,
my mind, like the sky, is clear.
All that matters is *this day.*

I choose *this day,*
my day to live fully.
All that matters is to be
in *this fullness.*

Being here and now is *everything.*

Today's Birthday

Billowy chalk-colored mist
rises from the surface of the water.
Fluffy smoke conceals life
moving on the distant bridge.

Mother Nature exhales.
The fog clears.
Cars and people emerge.
As she inhales,
they disappear again.

This life is far from where I sit.
It's like a dreamland or another planet.
I sense the shadowy movements
of those ghostly creatures from afar.
Reality distorted by the translucent screen
that divides here from there.

The cleansing mist moves diagonally
across the distant shoreline,
as it settles revealing vibrant shades
of azure and jade.

It is a rare gift to be in this morning,
as it is delivered from
behind the curtain of haze.

To witness the cleansing clouds
blanketing all things,
spreading, then dissipating,
rising then falling,
again and again,
from the water,
over the bridge,
onto the lake,
above the trees—

It's a cycle of continuous scrubbing,
clearing, and renewing,
breathing out and breathing in,
to bring forth the freshness of the new day.

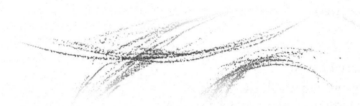

Surprise

My head lifts from the pillow,
feet touch the floor.
My mood still undeclared:
sunny or gloomy
elated or deflated
yet to be known—

The day is a neatly wrapped gift,
contents, *secret*, not ready to be revealed.

Time moves slowly.
My morning mind:
Clear.
Burdens of yesterday:
Gone.
Perceptions and possibilities:
Waiting to be born.

Life puts the artist's brush in my hand,
unwraps the blank canvas.
Images, shapes, palette—

I, choose the forms and colors
and when to unveil the gift,
The Masterpiece.

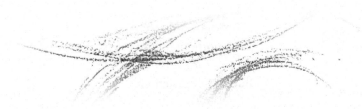

Sunlight Transformation

The veil lifts to reveal a brightly shining sun.
Green glows from bushes and trees,
transformed from gloomy grey.

Out of the overcast shadows of yesterday,
comes a golden sunrise.

Seeing this, I know
that out of these monotonous days,
the same brilliance will shine.

First as a tiny ray,
but then, just like the morning sun,
bursts of energy will ignite,
glowing, growing,
illuminating the Earth.

How quickly things can change—
First, in our mind's eye.
Then, in the universe.

How quickly things can change
when the sunlight comes out to greet us.

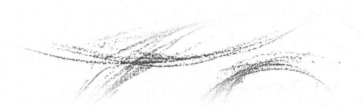

Chapter Three
Noticing

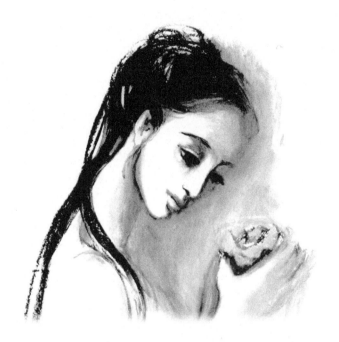

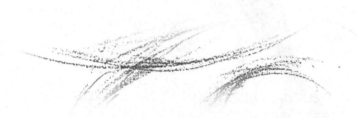

What I Miss

I walk in a trance,
unaware of the sights, smells, sounds,
and sensations of life right at my door.

Branches sway in the breeze.
Their tiny buds, not seen.
Their fragrant flowers, not smelled.
Fresh air blowing, not experienced.

Mind wrapped up in aimless wandering.

Newborn goslings silently chirp with
bodies waddling invisibly in single file.

Mind worrying about yesterday.

Fawn, left behind in the brush.
Why is my mother's heart not heavy?

Nature moves, breathes, flourishes, transforms—

All missed! Mind too stuck, anticipating tomorrow.

Stumbling on a rock,
I awaken and surrender,
abandon senselessness,
blindness, deafness.

My senses flooded,
life's abundance gushes in.

Nature's Moment

My friend, the squirrel stares at me from her home on the berm
above the beach.
> Raising up on her hind legs, she curiously tilts her head,
> pauses, and wonders why I am looking at her.

Waves rumble, as a fisherman wades into the water,
> his rod at attention,
> casting and pulling back.

Does he really want to catch a fish,
> or simply experience the day's intense beauty,
> and union with the water?

The tide churns, continuously rolling in.
> Aqua ripples melt into white foam,
> roaring, humming — one sound arises as another fades.

Multi-colored pigeons on a picnic table,
> befriend my campground neighbors.

White seagulls and black crows fly crisscross through blue skies,
> showing off their aviation skills.

Nature calls me to *this present moment,*
> of endless waters and brilliant sun,
> tempered just right by the breeze and clouds.

This moment of infinite awe, sound, and color.
The squirrel, fisherman, birds, and I,
all suspended in the endless wonders of nature.

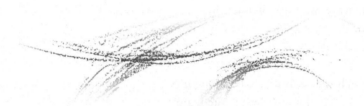

The Life of Geese and Cranes

Two pairs of geese and a pair of cranes come out on the lake to perform
their morning rituals.
Squawking, the geese mark their territory, warning others
not to invade.
The cranes stroll calmly along the shore, dipping their beaks
in and out of the water.
They search for tasty fish or bug treats, unaffected by the squawks
of the geese.

I sit on the dock and notice all the normalcy, the daily activities of geese
and cranes.
The morning sun warms me, and the cool breeze refreshes my body.
I'm surrounded by a symphony of sights, sounds and sensations.
The birds continue, unaware of what's going on in the outside world,
yet I, unlike them, am so shaken by these uncertain times.

I come to this place of refuge seeking peace.
In this moment, on the dock, I am free.
In this moment, there is no crisis.
There is no confusion or wondering.
There is no fear,
just the sunlight,
the breeze,
the geese,
the cranes—
and life just as it is.

Serenity Broken

Sitting in my usual spot by the lake:
crisp morning air invigorating,
sun kissing my cheeks,
the muscles of my face relax.

My nose awakens to the scent of dew:
eyes capture the reflections
of twinkling water,
ears feast on songs of birds.
Frogs accompany them
with a random tempo.
My senses, aroused,
softly energizing my soul.

Out of the calm,
mechanical sound intrudes:
a low monotonous hum
gradually intensifying.

A truck on the distant causeway—
engine reverberating
louder and louder.
Its penetrating moan
spreads over the water,
extinguishing other sounds.

My serenity completely shatters:
my face contracts,
brow furrows,
body tightens.
I hold my breath.

Ready to spring up,
the sound begins to fade.
The truck, bellowing grey exhaust,
pulls away across the causeway,
its echoes more and more distant.

My body relaxes.
Tension in my face releases
giving way to a gentle smile.
I sink back onto my cushion.

Once again, I can hear the birds,
enjoy the festival of sensations,
re-enter the comforting calm of my mindful state.

Funny how the full impact of this space,
was never so clear,
until lost for a moment
and now regained.

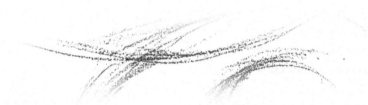

Nature's Symphony

Nature takes a deep breath
and exhales through puckered lips.
She flutters leaves as they cling to the baring branches.
One by one they dance to earth,
until the limbs are bare.

The evergreens sway as backup,
keeping rhythm for this visual symphony.
The smiling sun's warmth softens the discordant tempo,
transforming the notes into a brightly colored melody.

Night arrives, the curtain falls.
The symphony becomes silent.
Nature inhales and holds her breath.
In darkness she waits,
anticipating the concerto's next movement.

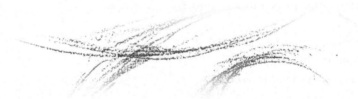

Cacophony of Birds

From silence comes the chirping of birds,
in different patterns and intonations.
I don't recognize their voices,
can't tell you their names,
or what they look like.
I don't even understand why birds tweet,
"Cheep—Cheep—Cheep."

Maybe I should "Google" that,
or even take up bird watching.
So like me, to move from pure experience,
to problem solving.

I remind myself,
it's not necessary to understand
the intimate facts or lives of birds,
to simply enjoy their chatter
and fully experience their wonder.

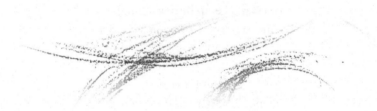

Fall Excursions

Arrive
Raindrops explode on the windshield,
sparkling as they collide and fade.
Wipers clear the debris.

Open
Sound of bacon sizzling,
aroma of coffee brewing.
First bite, first sip, energizing.

See
Pine needle lined trails like crisscross pick-up sticks.
Leaf showers gracefully cascade to Earth,
forming orange clusters on the shoreline.
They gaze like Narcissus at their twins on still waters.

Intertwine
Coast guard boats invade peaceful waters;
man superimposed on nature.
Vines creep and choke electric poles;
nature superimposed on man.

Release
Hiking: brisk steps, heart pumping,
muscles in relaxed contraction.
Nose tickled by the scent of burning leaves.
Cheeks kissed by the wind.

Choose
The indecisive movement of the seasons:
Starting, stopping, letting go.
I am *here*
as I move *there.*

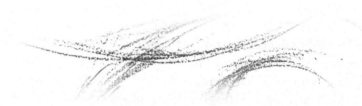

Rainbow Magic

There is a magical beauty to rainbows,

color vibrant — yet subdued,

Illuminating surroundings — yet transparent.

Infinitely spacious—no beginning — or ending.

You feel joy every time you see them.

You want to follow them,

all the while wondering where they go.

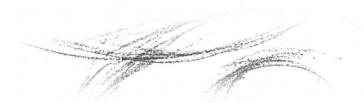

Chapter Four
Transforming

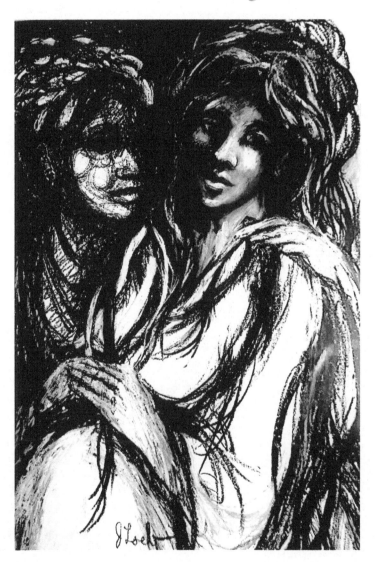

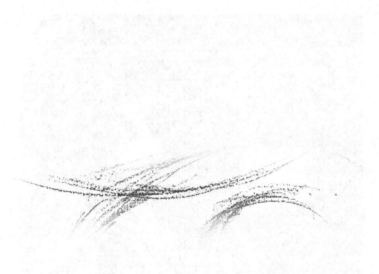

Shiny Objects

I'm floating in a sea of uncertainty
beneath the surface among shiny objects.
Reaching for one, I am distracted by another.
Turning back, the first one disappears.

Dazzled by yet another and another—
I try to scoop them up.
They slip through my looped arms,
gracefully dancing in slow motion,
just out of reach.

I turn and search, my goggles clouded.
I swim to the surface, gasping for air.
With one deep breath and not even a pause—
I dive down again and again.

Who Am I?

Looking out at an endless sky,
then zooming back into my own head,
I pause—
Walking out of my office for the last time,
I breathe in the fall air,
feel a new freedom—
No more "must do's" or "should do's!"

While drinking this morning's coffee,
I am unexpectedly stricken with a sense of loss.
Searching within, I ask:

Who am I?

Am I the baby born from my mother's womb,
the DNA of one woman and one man,
mixed in a unique combination to create this self?

Am I the tiny child awakening,
taking her first steps,
or uttering her first words,
giggling with these new-found superpowers?

Am I the straight A, B or C student,
struggling to overcome learning barriers—
dyslexic words on a page—
meeting with both failure and success?

Am I the young doctor making her first diagnosis,
or feeling the pain of life lost?

Am I the new mother, my babies moving in my belly,
holding them in my arms for the first time—
the sweetest, softest, warmest human experience?

Am I the wife, mother, bubby, grandma, leader, exercise junkie,
wannabe poet, meditator, motorhome mama?

Who am I?

These are all parts of me, my life's journey, yet not *all* of me.
My wholeness is not found in any one of these amazing experiences.

My true self is only revealed moving within
the limitless energy that runs through all of us,
flowing, intertwining with,
all spirits,
in all forms,
in all ways,
in all places—
even those we have yet to touch.

Ode to Freedom

Will I ever escape this self-imposed captivity?
I'm physically at home, but it feels like a cell.

It's not the configuration of these four walls,
but the configuration of my mind that binds me.

Does freedom come from our surroundings or from our souls?
Is the only way to experience freedom by opening our hearts
and quieting the constant chatter of our enslaving minds?

Where can one touch freedom?
In the vision of the stars, ocean, sky;
in each step taken on the earth,
or the scent of the flowers, the trees.

Must one hike up the highest mountain breathlessly,
walk on endless beaches until feet blister,
chasing the next more beautiful sunset,
travel to every corner of the universe,
searching for places that lived once
only in their imagination?

How does one find freedom? How do I?
I have looked in all these places:
the Alps of Switzerland,
the islands of Ecuador,
the Egyptian Pyramids,
bowing in temples to every God,
chasing Kiwis and Blue-footed Boobies,
whether in reality, or in my dreams.
But all this was to no avail,
The next day I was not free.

Close your eyes and travel the longest journey,
way down into your innermost soul,
beyond where your mind can reach.
Touch and accept the deepest part of your being.

Only there can you experience true freedom.
Only there can you be released,
to find a vastness, an openness,
that you have never known.

Travel there, my friend,
and you will be free.

Worlds Above and Below

Patches of wild swamp grass divide the cerulean waters,
dainty reeds of olive and khaki poke out in every direction.
Geese fly overhead in pairs,
flapping their wings and squawking to their partners,
as they awkwardly land on the bog.

My eyes feast on the sparkling lake,
endless skies and pine-lined shores—
sights and sounds all above the rim.

Gazing down to look beneath,
there lies a whole other world:
dark, cloudy, shadowy,
laced with velvety moss,
burnt umber rocks, and leafy red plants.

Minnows swim down,
tadpole bubbles float up.
Insects journey on blades of grass,
to bridge the worlds.

I stand on the dock taking the scene in.
How often does this deep exotic world go unnoticed?
Until today, I saw the upper world clearly,
yet failed to see the beauty just under the surface.

Brackish water parts.
An array of browns, reds, oranges, and yellows—
from dark to light—
invite me to dip my senses
into this stillness.
I wonder what it would be like to live
both above and below the surface?

How many times in life do we see only what lies above?
That which is in our line of vision, apparent to us, recognizable.
How many times in life do we fail to look into the murkiness?
Not seeing what lies deeper in places, people, things, experiences.
How many times in life are we deprived by our half-vision?

I peer through my multifocal lenses
to find the magic that only exists
when the two worlds merge into one.

Jumping In

The emerald and gold beetle grasps a blade of swamp grass,
trying to trick me into believing it's part of the greenery.
Its color and texture unmask the charade.

The bug clings tightly,
extremities and tentacles glued in place.
As the wind gusts and the grass sways,
the beetle remains motionless.

Like the bug, some people desire to blend in,
feel safe in their anonymity—
no one will notice or expect anything.
Like the beetle, they want to rest quietly,
be left alone to enjoy the breeze.

At any moment, a strong wind or gush of water
may seize the tiny insect's serenity.
The beetle, just like us, has no control over,
what happens in the unpredictable future?

What is the tiny insect or the tiny human to do?
Does it, do we, hold on more tightly?
Does it, do we, move slowly down the blade?
Does it, do we, dive into the water?
Or do we yield to indecisiveness,
hoping that if the wind is not too strong,
and the water is not too high, we will be, okay?

Now is the time to overcome hesitancy,
move to the bottom, jump into the water,
and confront the challenge.

Blindly clinging onto our blade of grass,
we never experience the full world.
Then when we least expect it,
we are washed into the water,
completely unprepared, swept away,
never knowing what hit us.

Mind Games

I struggle to let go of:
pervasive thoughts,
opportunities missed,
choices not made,
places not visited, driven past,
only to longingly admire them
in my rearview mirror.

If I stop, I still wonder:
Was the stay too short?
Were possibilities dismissed too soon?

I try to release:
regrets,
events that never happened,
circumstances not experienced,
things gone forever,
paths not taken,
risks avoided,
lives forsaken.
If they had happened, would this be so?

What creates this sense of longing?
Feeling the loss of things, I never possessed.
My mind, distracted, like on Mars,
yet body here, on Earth.
How do I come home?

Pause – Notice - Choose.
With eyes wide open,
I can see the wonder,
the newness on the horizon.
It's rising, it's here.
It can be lost in a blink.
If you lose your mind to things long gone,
you miss the joys of today.

My dears, there's no need for us to worry or regret.
We have the blessing, the gift of *now,*
born every day, hour, minute, second.
Put this book down immediately and live.

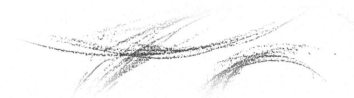

Chapter Five
Healing

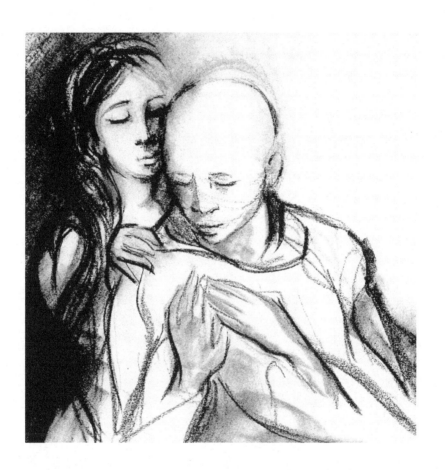

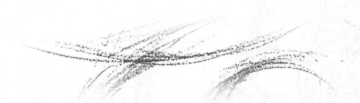

The Space Between

Time stops.
No sound, no motion.
Vision blurs.
Body, warm and tingling.
Suspended, I pause—

I breathe and travel deeper,
arriving in an unknown
yet familiar place—

Endless space opens.
Untethered, I float free—

From the source,
energy emerges:
calm, clarity, presence.
I step with intention
into today.

Opening the Heart

Somewhere deep within your heart,
there is a tiny door.
You have never ventured near,
nor dared to imagine opening it.
Traveling there is an arduous journey,
like sailing the seas in a hurricane,
climbing Everest in an avalanche,
swimming the channel in a straitjacket,
or finding your voice in a crowd of millions.

When you think of going there,
you whisper: *"I must not."*
For even more frightening,
is what lies beyond the door—
Thoughts, feelings, experiences,
left sleeping in the dark—
unknown.

Be brave, my loved one,
and hold my hand.
We will go there together.
And when the door, unlatched, swings open,
the clouds of all that frighten us,
will awaken and be set free:
floating, rising, dissipating.

Then revealed, will be, pure beauty,
soothing, comforting,
light and warm —
A tender spot within,
open and radiating,
with joy and love for all that is.

Beyond Words

Drawing back the curtain of words,

brilliant heart exposed,

pure expression flows.

Clarity which eludes the movement of lips,

contortions of tongue.

Aliveness that illuminates,

wordlessly penetrates.

Speaks in silence,

and sings the sentenceless song of eternity.

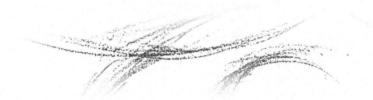

The Tree Within

There is a moment when
our bodies feel weak,
our minds are unsettled,
no firm ground to stand upon.

With each step, we are uprooted.
Waves of unsteadiness,
travel down our bodies.

In this moment,
we are filled with doubt.
"Can I move on?"

With stomachs queasy,
hands quivering,
we hold our breath.

This is when we should *breathe.*
For with each breath,
new energy arises,
awakening our minds,
with vision and clarity.

Strength emerges.
We stand erect, with presence,
like an ancient redwood.
Our souls empowered
and free
to enter *this day.*

The Lost Embrace / Found

(pandemic separation)

How can I hold you?
Awakening from dreaming,
the world seems so strange!
Who could have imagined?

I feel a hollowness in my chest,
my heart, my soul.
My arms longingly reach out
to touch emptiness.

How can I hold you, my child?
When you are so far away.
But even if you were close,
I couldn't, I shouldn't, embrace you—

I took so much for granted.
Now stripped away like a child ripped
from a mother's loving arms.
As she runs after the captors,
pleading and weeping,
she's thrown back.

How can I hold you, my little one,
in this moment, to fill this emptiness,
soothe this deep ache,
erase this sense of loss?
I took so much for granted.

Closing my eyes to see your warm smile,
then looking at your image on a screen.
Caressing your loving face with my eyes.
Hearing your gentle voice through devices.
The sound penetrates my inner being.

I remember your warmth,
the softness of your body,
and your childhood heartbeat.
I am in that moment.
I can even smell you.

How can I hold you, my loved one,
in this time of self-imposed separation?

Reaching deep within, I find you.
Sights, sounds, memories, senses.
awaken you within me.
It is not strange, but familiar.

We are part of the same life,
your being in my being,
always, united, even in adversity.
Together as one.

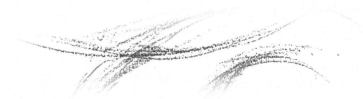

The Healing Moment:
The Healer Healed

Can you remember?
Can you feel it?
That moment when—
eyes met, hands touched, hearts united.

Data, remedies, treatments,
all fell away—

What remained was a deep connection,
a peaceful presence,
that filled our souls.

Knox

Taking second first steps…
   Eyes laugh, lips smile.
      Happy feet run on tiptoes
         to join the others.

      Not so long ago,
         stopped in his tracks.
            Loved ones, fearful.
               He, fearless.

            Tiny body without doubt.
               No worries, can'ts, won'ts,
                  only *why nots?*

               God's miracles do happen.
                  Taking second first steps...

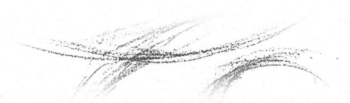

Epilogue

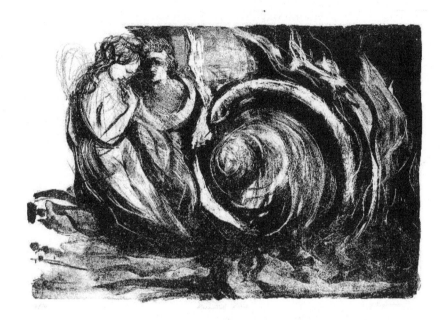

Humanity's Spring

Out of darkness and unknown places;
Out of months filled with loss, pain, uncertainty,
monotony that makes you scream;
Out of snowy, cloudy, rainy, days—
winds, chilling to the bones.

Out of waiting and waiting, driven to the edge
with deep wanting and even deeper fear,
stuck in your own tracks,
hesitant to take even one step.

A tiny flower bud appears hardly noticeable;
A woman walks her dog with a different cadence;
An unmasked couple with smiles set free,
yesterday revealed only in their eyes.

People pop out like the new growth of spring.
First, ever so slowly, then burst into blossom:
talking, laughing, walking, biking, running.
Folks sit on benches, on sand, on grass.
lay in hammocks, swing carefree.

Brightly colored beach umbrellas open,
vibrant layer after layer,
spreading shelter over life's picnic.
Juxtaposition of senses, sights, and sounds—
each experience more brilliant than the last.
Radiating energy and joy.

It is the spring of humanity—
life's ever renewing miracle
unexpectedly reborn to amaze us,
enfold us in wonder and freshness,
gently moving us,
once more into the light.

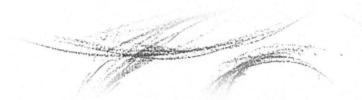

Appendix
Notes to the Reader

The Time of Words - 1968

Written by my teenage self when I first realized the power of words and self-expression through writing.

Chapter One: Grounding

Reflections on our roots, past generations and ancestors who ground us into the future.

To All Generations with Love - 2/29/2020

I attended a mindfulness retreat at Deer Park Monastery prior to the public acknowledgement of the pandemic. The dharma talk revolved around the idea that one hundred years from now, our names, voices, and faces will no longer be known by future generations, but the spirit and connection between all beings and things on the earth remain for eternity. The poem was written to send a message to all future generations that I will always be with them.

Judy Salsa's Tranquility Garden - written 8/1/2019 & revised 7/14/2021
My creativity is grounded in the rich gifts of my late mother. I only recently realized the depth of her influence. I dedicated a tranquility garden to her in 2019. Returning there during the pandemic I experienced a deeper sense of her creative spirit and revised this poem to reflect her eclectic inner beauty. This is illuminated further in the illustrations in this book, taken from her collection of artworks.

The Red Cardinal & *The Red Cardinal Returns* - 4/7/2020 & 5/9/2020

My father passed away from COVID-19 on April 7, 2020, on his 90th birthday. Minutes before his death, I saw a red cardinal outside my window that continued to return every day for weeks. I saw this as a message of comfort and a supporting presence.

We Never Know & *Coming Home* - 2/9/2021 & 2/14/2021

My mother-in-law died of a complication shortly after recovering from COVID-19. The last time we saw her, my husband paused and gently kissed her saying "I love you", not knowing she would die that same evening. I later recognized I was distracted and missed my own tender moment with her. This poem was written to remind us not to miss every chance we are given to experience such a moment. The second poem is a tribute to the freeing of her spirit. She had a strong faith in God. She loved purple and butterflies.

Chapter Two: Awakening

Celebrating the morning, renewal, possibilities, new times, and heralding in change.

Never-Ending Circle - 7/4/2021

Feeling the strong connection between myself, my daughters, and grandchildren, this poem expresses how we unite to travel through all of life's challenges while forever bound together by our love.

This Morning - 4/5/2020

An expression of joy and gratitude for a new day.

Today's Birthday - 5/23/2020[1]

Noting the cycle of the movement between the magical, refreshing, and renewing mist over the lake.

Surprise - 6/26/2020

Every morning there is a clean slate and an opportunity to create a day that is whatever you desire and decide to make it.

Sunlight Transformation - 4/26/2020

The pandemic brought many mornings that were filled with bad news and gloom, paired with unbearable monotony. I often called them "groundhog days", taken from the movie by the same name. On cloudy days, I noticed that when the sun came out, my mood was magically transformed from downtrodden to uplifted. This poem expresses a parallel between the clearing of overcast weather patterns, and the passing of heaviness of the pandemic on the world, and the belief that the metaphorical sun will come out to illuminate the earth.

---

[1] Kangaroo Lake, Door County, Wisconsin.

Chapter Three: Noticing

Appreciating and experiencing the richness of all things
as well as seeing nature and life through new eyes.

What I Miss - 5/9/2020[2]

Hiking in a nature preserve, I realized that my lack of attention so often caused me to miss the details of wondrous nature right in front of me.

Nature's Moment - 3/6/2020[3]

Camping along the California coast just after my mindfulness retreat and before the pandemic was declared publicly, I began consciously taking time to pause and notice the world around me. I developed a new appreciation for nature that continued to grow and heal me during the pandemic.

The Life of Geese and Cranes - 5/16/2021[4]

Sitting in the morning near the lake, I was in awe of how the daily activities of geese and cranes appeared completely unaffected by the pandemic. Even though the entire world may be in upheaval, we can benefit from finding space to alleviate the intensity of stark realities by living in the moment like these creatures of nature.

Serenity Broken - 8/1/2020[4]

Near the lake, my morning meditation was disrupted by the sound of a truck. I realized how I only appreciated this serenity when it was threatened. Sometimes, we don't fully appreciate things in our lives until we temporarily or even permanently lose them.

---

[2] Door County, Wisconsin.
[3] Carlsbad, California.
[4] Kangaroo Lake, Door County, Wisconsin.

Nature's Symphony - 11/2/2020

Watching a fall storm through my window, I noticed the harmonious movements of my backyard trees. I was able to visually experience melodies and rhythms.

Cacophony of Birds - 5/31/2020[5]

For the first time, I really noticed the intensity of the morning chirping of birds. I found myself trying to figure out the reasons for their morning sounds. On reflection, I dropped that idea to simply appreciate the richness of their voices.

Fall Excursion - 10/16/2020[6]

On a motorhome trip, a series of fall scenes juxtaposed with one another, captivated me with their vivid imagery.

Rainbow Magic - 3/23/2021

This poem is about the ethereal beauty of rainbows, how they make you feel and why you are drawn to them.

---

[5] Kangaroo Lake, Door County, Wisconsin.
[6] Lake Kentucky, Paris Landing State Park, Tennessee.

Chapter Four: Transforming

Searching deeper to discover one's true self.

Shiny Objects - 1/4/2020

So many times, I have been distracted by what can be referred to as "shiny objects", searching for the activity, mission, or teaching that will clarify my existence. This poem is a realization that even though this process may not be fruitful, my tendency is to keep searching and diving in.

Who Am I? - 4/29/2020

With a major shift in my career, I became distressed. Searching for a way to understand and explain my identity, this poem investigates elements of my past and present life as they define who I am. In the end, the wholeness of my true identity is found not in these external things but in my deeper soul.

Ode to Freedom - 5/6/2020

The poem examines what is true freedom and the external ways I have frantically tried to know and find it. I found the answer lies in a different place.

Worlds Above and Below - 5/21/2020[7]

Looking into the lake more deeply for the first time, I noticed the beauty below the surface. Drawing a parallel between this experience in nature and our lives, I wonder how often we fail to look beneath the surface in other aspects of our existence.

---

[7] Kangaroo Lake, Door County, Wisconsin.

Jumping In - 6/1/2020[8]

People often want to blend in, not leave their comfort zone and stay complacent. With the 2020 happenings; medically, socially, politically, and environmentally, I express how this may leave us unprepared to fall victim to unexpected, and unwanted consequences.

Mind Games - 5/2/2021

We often waste a lot of energy worrying about things we didn't do or things that didn't happen. In this process, we can miss the new opportunities of today.

---

[8] Kangaroo Lake, Door County, Wisconsin.

Chapter Five: Healing

Connecting with the healing energy that supports, nurtures, and mends us.

The Space Between - 2/22/2021

As we sit in silence, there is a sense of calm and openness that we can enter. We can feel suspended in time and space. This happens for me when I enter a meditative state.

Opening the Heart - 3/30/2020

As I began my healing journey, I was a little frightened to travel too deeply inward. When I found the courage to overcome this and let myself into my own soul, an indescribable energy and joy emerged.

Beyond Words - 2/27/2021

A dear friend of mine developed a brain tumor, which causes him, at times, to experience word block. I notice when he speaks from his heart, the intense clarity of his message magically comes through.

The Tree Within - 4/3/2020[9]

Trees have enduring strength combined with qualities of grounding, interconnection, and flexibility. Trees show us a powerful metaphor for strength that we can draw upon.

The Lost Embrace, Found - 4/25/2020

During the pandemic, I felt the deep separation and loss of not being able to embrace my children and grandchildren. Seeing my daughters' faces on Facetime, I reached deep inside my soul to find our spiritual bond that is beyond physical presence, and I found our deep connection.

---

[9] Kangaroo Lake, Door County, Wisconsin.

The Healing Moment: Healer Healed - *written 11/1/2020 & revised 4/14/2021*

The moments when I deeply connected with patients were the moments when I felt the clearest uplifting healing power. In the process of caring for them, I felt myself receiving a healing energy.

Knox - *6/22/2021*

On New Year's Eve 2020, my two-and-a-half-year-old grandson sustained a spinal cord injury. At first, he was completely paralyzed from the waist down. With God's grace, prayers, and his determination, (as   children are free of thoughts that he might not walk again) he began crawling, standing, walking, and finally running. It was truly God's Miracle.

Epilogue

Celebration that marks the exuberant release

as the pandemic burden lightened with new awareness emerging.

Humanity's Spring - *5/03/2021*
I experienced people joyfully coming to greet spring in Downtown Chicago. You could palpably feel a dwindling burden of the pandemic.

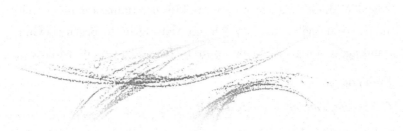

Acknowledgments

Daniel Goetschel: my husband for always being by my side, as we move through life's escapades together and for his careful reading of my book.

Daniel Friedland, MD: my friend, colleague and *Awakening Conscious Leadership* master for inspiring me daily as he shares his journey and legacy.

Shamash Alidina: my mindfulness teacher for imparting his wisdom and guidance at every turn. He instills me with the confidence (as well as a deadline) that made this book a reality.

Mary Thomson: my fellow mindfulness practitioner, and healthcare worker for her unconditional support, mindful listening, and insightful feedback.

Michael Krasner, MD & Ronald Epstein, MD, Co-founders and Co-leaders of *Mindful Practice,* **Frederick Marshall, MD,** Co-leader of *Mindful Practice:* for continuously showing me ways to cultivate greater levels of attentiveness, curiosity, beginner's mind, and presence in both my personal and professional life.

David Thoele, MD & Marjory Getz, PHD: the Co-founders of the *Advocate Aurora Narrative Medicine Group* for welcoming me into a community grounded in the principles of self-reflection, self-expression, and connection.

College of DuPage Writer's Workshop: my group members for their careful attention to my work in our weekly meetings and important feedback.

Georgia Casciato: my supporter and fellow health care advocate for her careful reading and kind editing suggestions.

MAVEN Project Community: the physician volunteers who support of practitioners in underserved clinics and the clinicians working in those settings for their purposeful work, collegiality, and fellowship.

———————————————

A special thanks to Mindful Practice, Teach Mindfulness and Narrative Medicine Groups, my family, and friends for always giving me their love and support during my great adventures.

My beloved Door County Wisconsin for providing me with a place of sanctuary, wondrous nature, and my mindful spot on North Kangaroo Lake.

About the Author

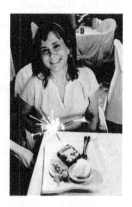

Barbara Loeb is a physician, poet, facilitator, and mentor who is committed to promoting healing, especially for those who care for others and often lose sight of their own need for nurturing. She was born and raised in an inner-city neighborhood on Chicago's Northside. She worked her way through Northwestern University and Rush Medical College.

For over 40 years, Barbara worked in numerous healthcare roles. First, as a primary care physician within her own Internal Medicine practice, and later, as a consultant sharing strategies to enhance physician-patient communication and connection. Finally, she served as a Chief Medical Officer navigating healthcare strategies within a variety of health organizations. She both observed and experienced the same challenges as her physician colleagues: fatigue, lack of self-care, and burnout. To provide herself with a greater measure of healing, she developed her own restorative ritual, which combines mindfulness, writing, and building deeper connections between patients and colleagues.

During the COVID-19 pandemic, for Barbara (as for so many others), the need for self-care became more urgent. In her first book *"How to Save a Life: Healing Power of Poetry"* written in 2020-2021, she utilizes the principles of presence, reflection, self-awareness, and compassion to create poetry that takes us along on her healer's journey. Her goal is to inspire her readers to reflect on their own path to well-being through self-expression. By sharing her poems and inner travels, she reveals the great strength that her readers can build through opening themselves and letting out their creative energy. She sends a message to future generations to connect to the grounding energy of the past. The volume is brilliantly illustrated with the artwork of her late mother Judy "Salsa" Loeb.

Barbara now spends her time writing and sharing what she has learned with clinician, caregivers, and others as they travel on their life journeys.

About the Artist

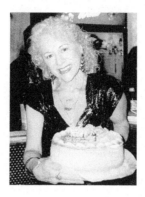

Judy "Salsa" Loeb was Born on March 18, 1931, to Eastern European Jewish immigrant parents. She grew up on the Westside of Chicago. She was a rebel in a time when women were discouraged from having a career. Despite this challenge, she found a way to attend the American Academy of Art.

As a young woman she traveled and performed in the Yiddish Theater. She married in 1951. When her two daughters were very young there was a hiatus in her work. As the girls entered school and after her marriage ended, her creative energy began to emerge once again.

Her early pieces were very realistic and primarily in oil. Later her style and mediums expanded to encompass semi-realistic and abstract images rendered in acrylic, conte crayon, oil-based crayon, mono-printing, and sculpture. Judy's work was heavily influenced by her study of Jungian Psychology with many archetypal images appearing in her art. Her subject matter reflected her many passions and life challenges; Salsa dancing, Tarot card reading, and the multiple roles and struggles experienced by women as mothers, lovers, daughters, and emerging individuals.

Judy left this world prematurely, suddenly in 1995.

She was the embodiment of creativity. In this book, her timeless images serve as a window inviting you to see the richness in your own soul. The hope is that this will inspire you to release the creativity that wants to emerge from within.

Made in the USA
Coppell, TX
24 December 2021

69972781R10066